HOW TO READ AN ECG

Basic interpretation for nurses and other health workers

HOW TO READ AN ECG

Basic interpretation for nurses and other health workers

REVISED EDITION

by Margaret G. Blowers, R.N., B.S.N.
and Roberta J. Smith, R.N., M.Ed.

Medical Economics Company **MEBD** Book Division
Oradell, New Jersey 07649

and

Delmar Publishers
Albany, New York 12205

ISBN 0-87489-137-X

Medical Economics Company
Oradell, New Jersey 07649

ISBN 0-8273-1307-1

Delmar Publishers
Albany, New York 12205

Printed in the United States of America

First Edition   May, 1973
Fifth Printing   March, 1976
Revised Edition   June, 1977
Second Printing   October, 1978

Contents

Publisher's Notes

This revised and expanded edition of the original book from RN Magazine by Herbert H. Butler, M.D., is the result of a conscientious team effort by the two authors.

MARGARET G. BLOWERS, R.N., B.S.N., is an instructor in intensive coronary and respiratory nursing care, in courses given by the Continuing Education Department of Hackensack Hospital, Hackensack, N.J. She is a graduate of the Frances Payne Bolton School of Nursing of Western Reserve University in Cleveland, Ohio, and of Seton Hall University in South Orange, N.J.

ROBERTA J. SMITH, R.N., M.Ed., is an instructor in intensive coronary care at Hackensack Hospital. She also teaches an ECG/arrhythmia course for R.N.s at Bergen Community College, Paramus, N.J. She is a graduate of St. Luke's Hospital Nursing School, Bethlehem, Pa.; Cedar Crest College, Allentown, Pa.; and Lehigh University, Bethlehem, Pa.

JO ANNE CASSELLA of Medical Economics Company's art department is responsible for the typography and design of the book.

Introduction

Thousands of heart patients are being saved in hospitals today because of the prompt assessment and treatment of cardiac arrhythmias by nurses and other trained emergency personnel. Usually it is the nurse who is at the patient's side when such a catastrophe occurs, and it is the nurse who has been mostly responsible for the marked decrease in cardiac mortality in coronary- and intensive-care units. Physicians with little or no experience in electrocardiography look to nurses with special knowledge for interpretation of electrocardiograms.

Since lethal arrhythmias also occur outside the critical-care units, all nurses need to have some basic knowledge of the electrocardiogram and, at the least, be able to recognize the very dangerous cardiac abnormalities. The same is true for other emergency personnel, ambulance attendants, and police.

Recognition of a dangerous arrhythmia—particularly through alert observation of an abnormal ECG—can considerably improve a patient's chance for survival. This book focuses on the basic knowledge needed about (1) the normal ECG, (2) noncatastrophic arrhythmias, and (3) life-threatening arrhythmias and the treatment measures that can be instituted to correct them.

Diagrams of the electrical activity of the heart and representative ECG patterns are presented to help the reader differentiate between what may be a simple cardiac problem and a potentially dangerous one. With a little bit of background and experience, emergency personnel, including R.N.s, can learn to recognize almost all life-threatening arrhythmias so that they can initiate treatment or call on more experienced help.

Treatment must be based on a combination of: comprehensive knowledge of the effect of arrhythmias, clinical information about the individual patient's condition, and awareness of legal limitations imposed by the institution or local government.

Introduction

Glossary

Aberrant. Wandering from the normal course.

Antiarrhythmia drugs. Those commonly administered to counteract irregularities in cardiac rate or rhythm.

Arrhythmia. A cardiac rhythm disturbance due to a dysfunction in impulse formation or conduction.

Atrium. One of the upper chambers of the heart.

Automaticity. The ability of the myocardial cells to discharge an electrical impulse.

Bundle of His. Small band of cardiac muscle fibers that disperse the atrial contraction consistently to the ventricles.

Cardiac arrest. Ventricular standstill. The heart stops beating and death can occur in one to three minutes.

Cardioversion. A synchronized electrical shock timed so that it does not occur during the vulnerable period of the T wave.

Coronary arteries. Small vessels that originate from the aorta above the aortic valve and provide the blood supply to the heart.

Defibrillation. Electrical shock not timed to the cardiac cycle. It depolarizes all fibrillating myocardial cells simultaneously, allowing the SA node to resume pacing.

Depolarization. Condition in which the electrical impulse arrives from the SA node, the permeability of the cell membrane is changed, and the polarity of the cell reverses.

Ectopic. Beat arising from a focus outside the sinus node.

Electrocardiogram. A graphic recording of the electrical activity produced by the heart muscle.

Electrodes. Contacts attached to designated points on the limbs and chest wall of the patient that record electrical impulses of the heart and transmit them to a graphic recorder.

Extrasystole. Systole originating outside the sinus node; a premature beat usually bears this label.

2

Fibrillation, ventricular. Condition in which the electrical activity and ensuing ventricular contraction is disorganized, and the heart quivers erratically.

Heart block (complete). Condition which results when conduction is blocked by a lesion at any level in the AV junction.

Hypoxia. Oxygen deficiency.

Ischemia. Deficiency of blood supply to tissue because of arterial constriction or obstruction.

Isoelectric. Neither negative nor positive electrical potential; giving off no current. The ECG inscribes a straight line.

Joule. Unit of energy equivalent to 1 watt-second.

Myocardial infarction. Occlusion of a coronary artery that causes blocking of the blood supply to the heart muscle, severe ischemia, and destruction of tissue.

Pacemaker (physiological). The SA node, which sends out regular impulses to stimulate the myocardium.

Parasympathetic nervous system. Acts to slow the heart rate.

PAT. Paroxysmal atrial tachycardia.

Patient monitor oscilloscope. A device that shows electrical activity of the heart on a screen; it is not a permanent record unless it has a strip record attached.

Precordial ECG waves. Those emanating from chest leads.

Preexcitation. Premature activation of a portion of the ventricle.

P wave. As shown on the ECG, it represents the electrical impulse going through the atria.

PVC. Premature ventricular contractions (dangerous when they hit the T wave because a death-producing arrhythmia may result). Also called **PVD,** premature ventricular depolarization.

QRS complex. The letters have no specific meaning; Q, R, and S waves represent the electrical impulse going through the ventricle.

Refractory. Not responsive to stimuli or treatment.

Repolarization. Condition in which the electrical potential returns to the normal (resting) state.

SA node. Normal physiological pacemaker.

Sick sinus syndrome. Term used to indicate a failing sinus node, seen as severe slowing, blocking, or arresting of the SA node, or as an alternating sinus tachycardia-sinus bradycardia pattern.

Supraventricular. Above the ventricles.

Sympathetic nervous system. Acts to increase the heart rate.

Systole. Contraction phase of the cardiac cycle.

Vector. An electrical force of a known magnitude and direction.

Ventricles. Lower chambers of the heart with thick, muscular walls.

Watt-second. Unit of electrical energy equal to wattage x time in seconds. (see Joule.)

HOW TO READ AN ECG

Normal ECG and related heart anatomy

The electrocardiogram presents a visible record of the heart's electrical activity by means of a stylus that traces the activity on a continuously moving strip of special paper.

Normal ECG

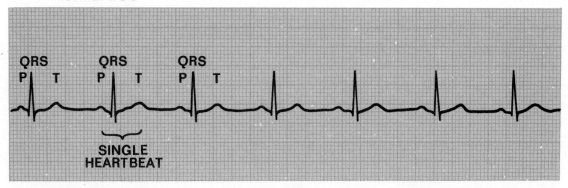

Normal ECG. All beats appear as a similar pattern, equally spaced, and have three major units: P wave, QRS complex, and T wave.

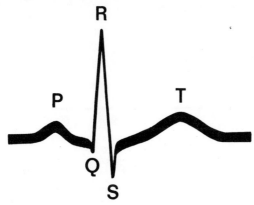

Normal single heartbeat. Each beat manifests as five major waves: P, Q, R, S, and T. The Q, R, and S all represent the same part of the heart (ventricle). They are usually referred to as a unit: the QRS complex.

The heart in relation to the ECG

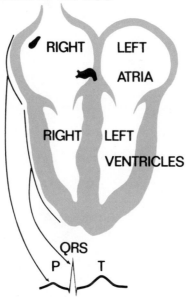

The heart in relation to the ECG. Each wave represents transmission of an electrical impulse through the heart muscle (depolarization), which causes the muscle to contract and thus eject blood. The P wave reflects the impulse going through the atria. The QRS complex reflects the impulse going through the ventricles. The T wave is produced by the electrical recovery (repolarization) of the ventricles.

Depolarization. As the electrical impulse moves across the cells of the myocardium, the polarity (negative or positive electrical charge) of the cells is changed.

The resting cell has a negative charge:

The electrical impulse carries a positive charge into the cell changing the polarity:

This is called depolarization:

It is followed by a continuing wave of repolarization which restores the cell to its original charge:

The cell is then ready to receive another stimulus.

Normal electrical pathway

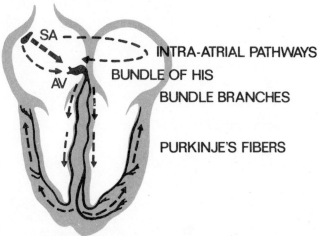

SA

INTRA-ATRIAL PATHWAYS

AV

BUNDLE OF HIS

BUNDLE BRANCHES

PURKINJE'S FIBERS

Normal electrical pathway. The impulse originates and is conducted to the muscle cells by way of specialized tissue that has automaticity and conductivity. All myocardial tissue has these properties, but they are developed to a greater degree in the conduction system.

The electrical impulse originates in the sinoatrial (SA) node—the normal physiological pacemaker—located near the top of the right atrium. The impulse spreads through intra-atrial pathways to the atrioventricular (AV) node located at the junction of the atria and ventricles. After a brief delay, the impulse continues through the bundle of His, the right and left bundle branches, Purkinje's fibers, and finally activates the ventricular muscle cells. Both the SA and AV nodes are innervated by the sympathetic system which increases the heart rate, and by the parasympathetic system (vagus nerve) which slows the rate.

The SA node normally discharges impulses at a rate of 60-100 times per minute, AV junctional tissue at 40-60, and Purkinje's fibers at 20-40. The pacemaker firing at the fastest rate controls the heartbeat. This

6

property of multiple pacemakers provides a reserve or backup system against cardiac arrest.

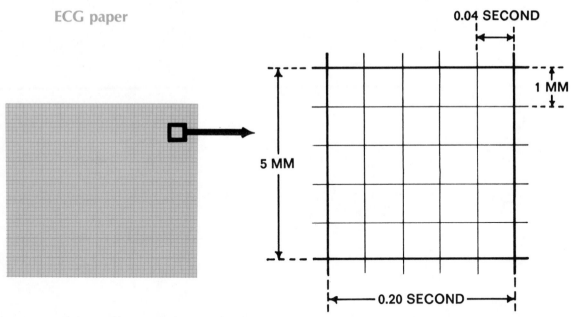

ECG paper. To understand the significance of each wave and interval, we need to know the significance of the small and large blocks on the ECG paper. The paper moves through the ECG machine at the rate of 1 inch per second (standard setting). One small block represents 0.04 second on the horizontal line and 1 mm. on the vertical line. Since a large block is five small blocks wide and five high, each large block represents 0.20 second (horizontal) and 5 mm. (vertical).

Now that we know these basic measurements and are familiar with the relation of the ECG waves to the heart anatomy, let's discuss the significance of each wave and interval:

P wave

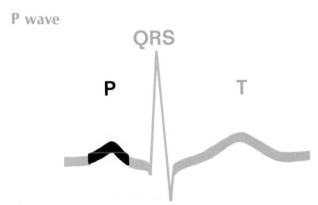

The **P wave** is the first upward deflection and represents the atrial depolarization. Enlargement of the P wave might occur in such condi-

7

tions as mitral stenosis or chronic obstructive pulmonary disease, which would cause atrial hypertrophy. The P wave is usually considered enlarged if it is more than three small blocks (3 mm.) high and/or three small blocks (0.12 sec.) wide.

PR interval

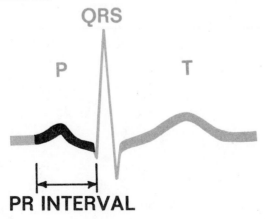

The **PR interval** extends from the beginning of the P wave to the onset of the Q wave. It represents conduction of the impulse through the atria and into the AV node. Lengthening occurs when the impulse is forced to travel at a slower rate, a condition occurring in the presence of arteriosclerosis, inflammation, insufficient oxygen supply, or scarring from rheumatic heart disease. It can also occur as an effect of such drugs as digitalis. The normal PR interval covers no more than five small blocks (0.20 second).

QRS complex

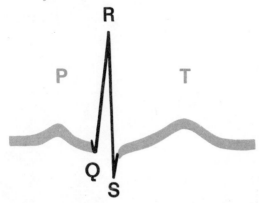

The **QRS complex** consists of three deflections: Q wave, the first downward stroke; R wave, the first upward deflection; and S wave, the downstroke following the R wave. Not every QRS complex shows a discrete Q, R, or S wave, but the configuration is still referred to as the

8

QRS complex to denote a ventricular impulse. An enlarged Q wave (greater than a small square) may indicate a myocardial infarction. An enlarged R wave usually indicates enlarged ventricles. The normal duration of the QRS is less than three small blocks (0.12 second).

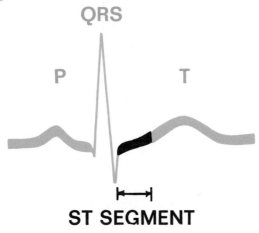

ST SEGMENT

The **ST segment** begins at the end of the S wave (the point where the line turns right) and ends at the beginning of the T wave. It is elevated in an acute myocardial infarction or muscle injury. It is depressed when the heart muscle isn't getting a sufficient supply of oxygen—for example, during an episode of angina or coronary insufficiency. It may sag as an effect of digitalis. ST changes are usually transient.

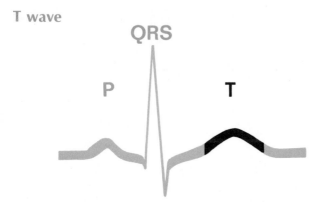

The **T wave** represents electrical recovery of the ventricular contraction. (The electrons are in the process of moving back into the normal resting position.) The T wave is flat or inverted in response to position change, food intake, or certain drugs. It may be elevated when the serum potassium is elevated. The normal T wave is no more than 10 small blocks (10 mm.) high in the precordial (chest) leads and five small blocks (5 mm.) in the remaining leads.

U wave

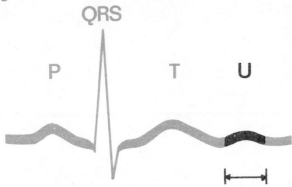

The **U wave** is a small upward deflection following the T wave. It is seldom present but may occur when the serum potassium level is low.

The ECG leads

It is assumed that the reader has some knowledge of what the ECG leads look like and how they are placed. Here we will review briefly some terminology and basic concepts necessary to an understanding of our discussion of the ECG. To take a routine ECG, 12 leads are used:

On the limbs: I, II, III, AVR, AVL, AVF

On the chest: V_1, V_2, V_3, V_4, V_5, V_6

Each lead records the same electrical impulse on the ECG but from a different position in relation to the heart. Each can be read separately, or they can be read in combination.

The limb leads show the current flow from one area of the body toward another. Lead I shows electrical activity from the right arm to the left arm, Lead II from right arm to left leg, and Lead III from left arm to left leg. The right-leg position is not displayed as part of the flow of current through the heart, as it is used for grounding the system.

The abbreviation AVR stands for augmented vector right, an added point of reference for diagnosis. AVL and AVF represent the left side and foot positions, respectively.

In diagnosing arrhythmias, Lead II and the right-chest leads are commonly used because they most consistently show an easily visible P wave. Many times, the P wave provides the key to success in determining the identity of an arrhythmia.

The most important leads to remember in relation to the anatomy of the heart are:

V_1, AVR	Right side of heart
V_2, V_3, V_4	Transition between right and left sides of heart

10

V₅, V₆, I, AVL   Left side of heart

II, III, AVF   Inferior heart

By knowing what part of the heart each lead represents, one can localize the area of pathology shown on the ECG. For example: If an infarct shows up on Leads II, III, and AVF only, it is located in the inferior aspect of the heart.

Limb leads

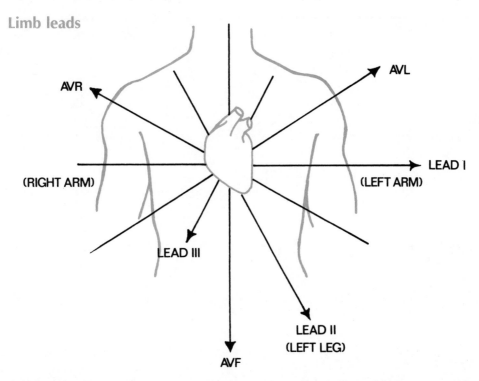

If **limb leads** are shown as crossing the chest over the heart on the frontal plane, they normally represent the above vectors.

Precordial (chest) leads

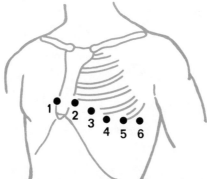

The **precordial leads** provide points of reference across the chest wall as illustrated.

Format for analyzing arrhythmias

Normal sinus rhythm

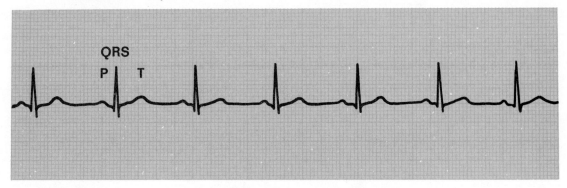

If all findings are normal, **normal sinus rhythm** is present.

Rhythm. Regularity may be determined using calipers or any determinant which would represent a fixed interval for comparison.

Determining the cardiac rate

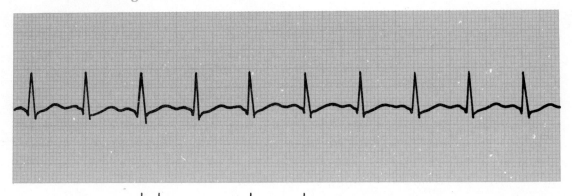

⊔   **⌴_____⌴**
1 LARGE BLOCK   **3 LARGE BLOCKS BETWEEN EACH QRS COMPLEX**

Alternate methods of **determining the cardiac rate.** 1. Since each large block on the ECG paper represents 0.20 second, 300 large blocks represent 1 minute (.20 x 300 = 60 seconds). To get a rough but quick cardiac rate determination, count the large blocks between each R wave (QRS complex) and divide 300 by this figure. In the example above, there are three large blocks between each R wave. Dividing 300 by 3 gives us a rate of 100 beats per minute. (If there were two blocks, the rate would be 150 beats; four blocks, 75 beats.) **or:** 2. Count the number of complexes in a 6-inch strip and multiply by 10 (useful for irregular rhythms). **or:** 3. Use a prepared rate table or ruler.

ECG characteristic	Normal finding
Rhythm	Regular (distance between QRS complexes varies by no more than three small squares)
Rate	60-100 beats per minute (3-5 large squares between QRS complexes)
P wave	Present and upright All shaped alike
PR interval	P wave precedes QRS Duration greater than three but less than five small squares (0.12-0.20 sec.) Time interval is same for all beats
QRS complex	Present All shaped alike Duration not more than three small squares (0.12 sec.)

Sinus arrhythmias

Pathway of sinus rhythms. Three arrhythmias that originate in the SA node are sinus arrhythmia, sinus tachycardia, and sinus bradycardia. The path of their electrical impulses is exactly the same as that of normal sinus rhythm. Because of this, the P wave, the PR interval, and the QRS complex have the same configuration as the normal rhythm. The difference lies in the regularity and the rate of the impulses.

Sinus arrhythmia

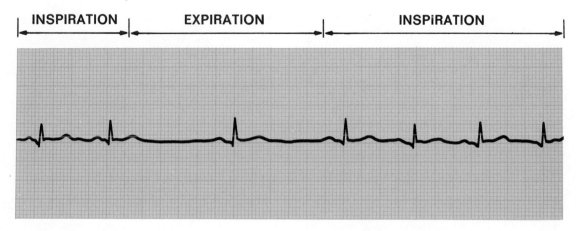

| INSPIRATION | EXPIRATION | INSPIRATION |

Sinus arrhythmia. All complexes are normal, but the heart rhythm is irregular. The rate increases with inspiration, decreases with expiration. This irregularity is common in children and may occur in adults in relation to certain respiratory patterns. It does not decrease cardiac output and does not lead to more serious arrhythmias.

Sinus tachycardia

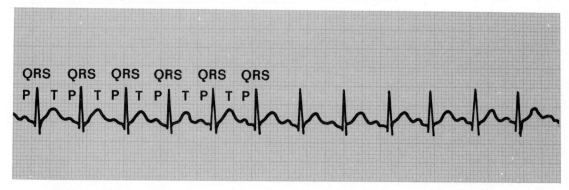

Sinus tachycardia. All complexes are normal, but the heart rate is more than 100. (It seldom exceeds 150.) Excessive sympathetic nerve stimulation causes the increased rate. Common causes are physical activity, anxiety, and fever. An increased rate may also be a compensatory response to decreased cardiac output.

Since sinus tachycardia is usually secondary to factors outside the heart, the treatment is directed to the underlying cause. No cardiac drugs are necessary.

Sinus bradycardia

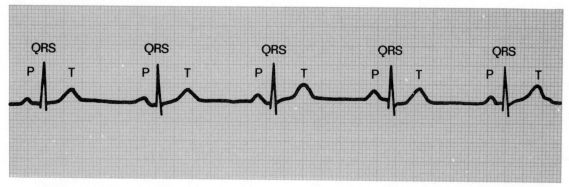

Sinus bradycardia. This arrhythmia is defined as a heart rate below 60 while all complexes remain normal. Sinus bradycardia is seen as an expected manifestation in well-trained athletes. It may occur in patients on digitalis, morphine, or pressor amines (for treatment of low blood pressure). A significant slowing may cause a decrease in cardiac output which could lead to cerebral or coronary insufficiency. An

additional hazard is that bradycardia may permit other ectopic foci to take over, causing serious arrhythmias.

The decision to treat sinus bradycardia is based on an evaluation of the patient's clinical picture. If drug therapy is indicated, I.V. atropine is often used to inhibit the vagus (heart-slowing) nerve, thus speeding up the heart rate. If atropine is not successful, isoproterenol (Isuprel) in 5% glucose solution may be administered. While this solution is running, it is important to watch the ECG monitor for signs of a dangerously rapid ventricular rate. If the patient does not respond satisfactorily, use of an electrical pacemaker may be necessary.

Sinus block

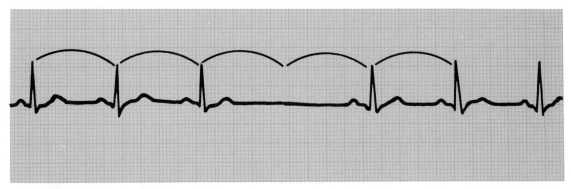

Sinus block occurs when a beat is not transmitted out of the SA node. No P, QRS, or T is present at the cycle interval for one or more beats.

Sinus arrest

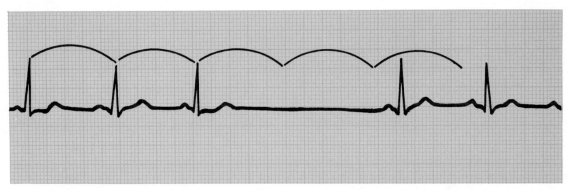

Sinus arrest occurs when the SA node fails to send out an impulse for a period of time. This interval between beats is not a multiple of the heartbeat cycle length.

If either event produces symptoms of cerebral insufficiency, treatment (atropine, isoproterenol, or a pacemaker) is indicated.

HOW TO READ AN ECG

PART II
Atrial arrhythmias   Page 16
Junctional (nodal) arrhythmias Page 21

Atrial arrhythmias

Portions of atrial tissue may become excitable and initiate impulses. These ectopic foci will control the heartbeat if they occur at a rate faster than impulses from the SA node.

ECG for PAC

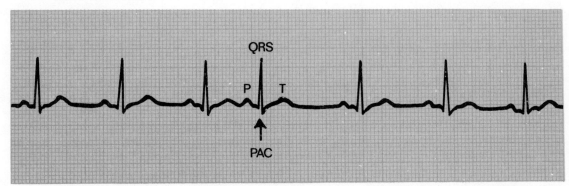

Premature atrial contraction (PAC) is a beat initiated by an ectopic atrial focus and appearing early in the cycle (before the next expected

sinus beat). Since the impulse arises from a site other than the sinus node, the shape of the P wave and the length of the PR interval may be different. The premature P wave is sometimes difficult to distinguish when it is superimposed on the preceding T wave.

This PAC is usually conducted through the ventricular pathway in the normal manner not affecting the shape of the QRS. A pause will follow the PAC, and the SA node will start a new cycle of sinus beats.

The significance of PACs is that they indicate atrial irritability. Frequent PACs may be warnings of more serious atrial arrhythmias and are usually treated. Quinidine is often the drug of choice.

ECG for PAT

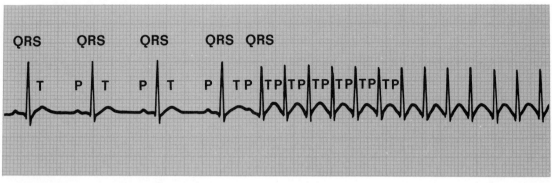

NORMAL SINUS RHYTHM   ↑ ONSET OF PAT

Paroxysmal atrial tachycardia (PAT) is an abrupt episode of tachycardia with the heart rate usually between 140-250 beats per minute, averaging about 180. The pacemaker site is an ectopic atrial focus. As with a PAC, the P wave may be abnormally shaped, or not seen because it is buried in the preceding T wave. The QRS appears normal.

PAT may be seen in young adults with normal hearts or in individuals with organic disease. The patient frequently complains of a sudden pounding or fluttering in the chest associated with weakness or breathlessness.

The fast rate stresses the heart and increases its need for oxygen. Tachycardia may also diminish cardiac output because of shortened ventricular filling time. The heart is beating so rapidly that the ventricle does not have time to fill completely. Therefore, each beat pumps out less blood. In a relatively asymptomatic and stable patient, sedation and calming measures may be sufficient. If PAT persists, the usual treatment is to stimulate the vagus nerve. That slows the heart rate. The physician may accomplish this by carotid sinus massage. Since this can produce dangerous slowing or cardiac arrest, the patient should be monitored and resuscitation equipment readily available.

Other measures which stimulate the vagus nerve include: gagging

the patient with a tongue blade, stimulating the anal sphincter with a rectal thermometer or tube, and applying pressure to the eyeball. A Valsalva maneuver (forced expiration against a closed glottis) will increase intrathoracic pressure, decrease venous return, raise the blood pressure, and slow the pulse.

If the patient is not hypertensive, drugs such as metaraminol (Aramine) I.V. in 5% glucose in water may be given slowly. The rise in blood pressure will stimulate the vagus. A parasympathetic drug, edrophonium chloride (Tensilon), 5-10 mg. I.V. slowly, also is useful, provided no hypotension or chronic lung disease coexists.

Conduction-depressing drugs such as digitalis, propranolol (Inderal), and procainamide (Pronestyl) may also slow the heart rate. If the patient is receiving digitalis, observe closely for excessive depression of impulse conduction.

When the heart continues to beat rapidly for a period of time, a synchronized electrical shock (cardioversion) is used by some doctors to prevent heart failure.

ECG for PAT with block

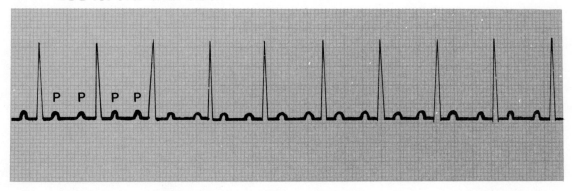

Most cases of PAT exhibit no block, and all the impulses are transmitted by the AV node to the ventricles. Occasionally, some beats are not conducted to the ventricles—a condition called **PAT with block.** The atrial rate is 140-250 and the ventricular rate is slower. This is frequently seen as a result of digitalis toxicity.

Atrial flutter. As the name implies, atrial flutter is a rapid, regular fluttering of the atrium. It usually occurs in a pathologic heart (usually arteriosclerotic or rheumatic), in contrast to PAT, which is usually associated with a normal heart. The P waves take on a saw-toothed appearance because they are coming from a focus other than the sinus node at a very rapid rate. Like PAT, the impulse comes from one ectopic focus in the atrium. Unlike PAT, the atrial rate (not pulse or ventricular rate) is between 250 and 350 per minute compared to the PAT average atrial rate of about 180 per minute. Although the following rules are oversimplified, they are helpful in distinguishing the atrial

arrhythmias from each other:
1. The atrial rate in sinus tachycardia goes up to 150/minute.
2. The atrial rate in PAT is between 140-250/minute.
3. The atrial rate in atrial flutter is between 250-350/minute.

ECG for atrial flutter

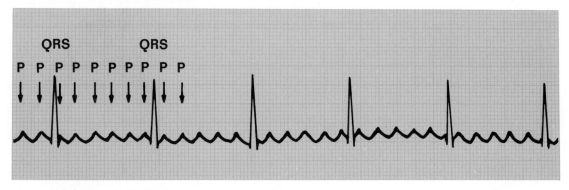

ECG for atrial flutter. The arrows indicate the P waves that are coming from the fast ectopic focus in the atrium. Notice that not every P wave stimulates a QRS complex. Since the abnormality is above the AV node, the QRS complexes that appear are normal in configuration.

Because the P waves are coming so rapidly, the AV node cannot accept and conduct each one, and therefore some degree of blockage occurs at the node. For example: If the atrial rate is 300, the ventricular rate (same as the pulse rate) may be 150. The block is thus said to be 2:1, since there are two atrial impulses per one ventricular response. In the diagram, five or six P waves precede each QRS.

Treatment of atrial flutter is indicated if the ventricular rate is sufficiently rapid to be potentially dangerous to the patient.

Classical initial treatment of atrial flutter has always been digitalization. Digitalis slows the pulse by blocking the AV node so that fewer P waves are conducted to the ventricles. A fast cardiac rate is relatively ineffectual and can lead to congestive heart failure. For this reason some doctors do not digitalize but go directly to cardioversion.

Sometimes as a result of digitalis therapy, a very slow ventricular rate may develop and will need treatment.

Atrial fibrillation is a very fast atrial rate arising from many ectopic foci. There is an irregular ventricular response, normal P waves are replaced by irregular rapid waves, and the total atrial configuration may resemble a wavy baseline or almost straight line.

These P waves (often called fibrillatory waves) assume different shapes because they are coming from different foci in the atrium. In contrast, the P waves in atrial flutter are regular and uniform because they are coming from one focus.

19

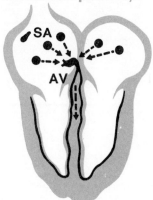

Normal pathway   **Atrial fibrillation pathway**

SA   AV   SA   AV

Since P waves in atrial fibrillation are not clearly discernible, the atrial rate cannot be measured but is much faster than the ventricular rate. With no definite P waves, no PR interval can be determined. The ventricular rate may be fast or slow but is usually irregular.

ECG for atrial fibrillation

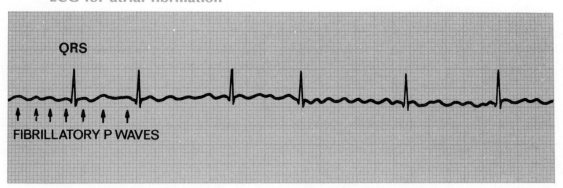

QRS

FIBRILLATORY P WAVES

ECG for atrial fibrillation. This is usually seen in older patients with arteriosclerotic or rheumatic heart disease. These conditions lead to scarring of the atrium, which disrupts the normal course of the P wave.

The treatment depends on the patient's clinical condition, cardiac rate, and drug status. As the cardiac rate increases above 100, cardiac output becomes less and less because the heart has less time to fill with blood. Many patients with atrial fibrillation are in congestive failure and have a rapid cardiac rate. They may benefit from digitalis, which strengthens contractions and slows the ventricular rate.

If atrial fibrillation is a life-threatening emergency, cardioversion may be instituted, starting with 50-100 watt-seconds. But cardioversion is dangerous if the patient is on digitalis, for the drug predisposes the heart to lethal arrhythmias after an electrical shock. The risk of arrhythmia increases as the number of watt-seconds is increased.

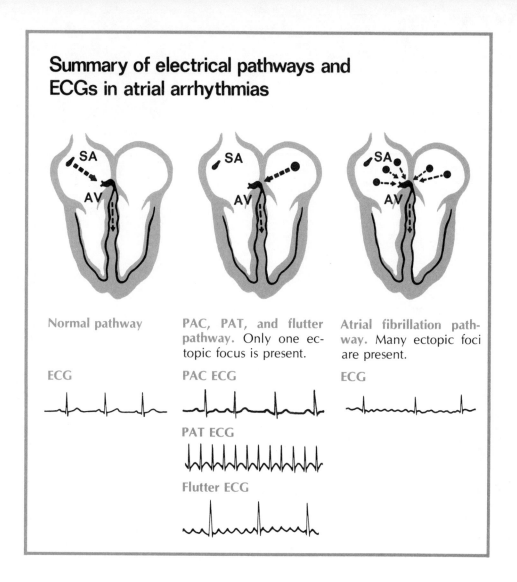

Summary of electrical pathways and ECGs in atrial arrhythmias

Normal pathway

ECG

PAC, PAT, and flutter pathway. Only one ectopic focus is present.

PAC ECG

PAT ECG

Flutter ECG

Atrial fibrillation pathway. Many ectopic foci are present.

ECG

Junctional (nodal) arrhythmias

After the cardiac impulse has traversed the atria, it reaches the atrio-ventricular junction (AV node). The AV node acts as a gateway to the conduction system that penetrates the dense muscular tissue of the ventricles. Its usual function is to receive the impulse, delay it for an instant, and then conduct it to the ventricular pathway. Junctional tissue in the area of the AV node also has the capacity to initiate impulses at the rate of 40-60 times per minute, and can act as a backup system if the sinus node fails to fire. In conditions of disease or anoxia, the tissue can become irritable and initiate rapid ectopic impulses.

Normal pathway Junctional pathway

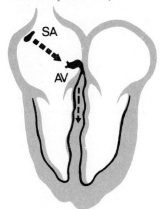 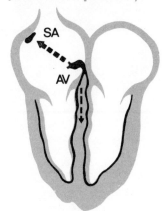

When an impulse arises in the junctional area, it will activate the atria through retrograde (backwards) conduction, causing the P wave to be inverted (in leads where the P would normally be upright). The impulse will be conducted through the ventricular pathways in a normal manner and thus the QRS will be normal.

The inverted P wave appears directly before, buried in, or directly after the QRS complex, depending on whether the atrium or the ventricle is activated first.

Junctional complexes

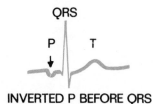 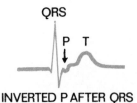

INVERTED P BEFORE QRS   P HIDDEN IN QRS   INVERTED P AFTER QRS

Junctional premature contraction (JPC)

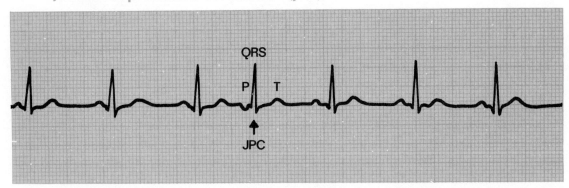

A **junctional premature contraction (JPC)** is an ectopic beat that arises from tissue in the junctional area and appears before the next expected sinus beat. The P will be inverted before or after the QRS, or may be

completely hidden in the QRS. A JPC can be distinguished from a PAC by the appearance of the P wave.

Infrequent JPCs do not require treatment. Frequent JPCs indicate tissue irritability and may be treated with a myocardial depressant.

Junctional rhythm

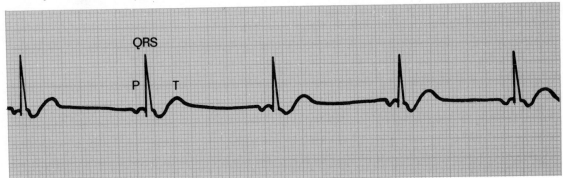

Junctional rhythm occurs when the pacemaker site is junctional tissue. The characteristic rate is 40-60 beats per minute, but this may be accelerated to the range of tachycardia. The rhythm will consist of repeated, regular junctional complexes.

Junctional rhythm may occur as a transient condition when the SA node is inadequate. It may also occur as a result of toxicity from digitalis or other myocardial depressants. Treatment, if necessary, depends on the cause of the rhythm and the effect of the rate on the patient's clinical condition.

Junctional tachycardia

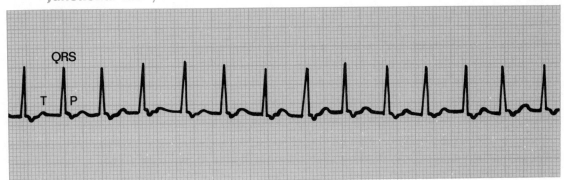

Junctional tachycardia is a junctional rhythm with a rate of 100-180 beats per minute.

This arrhythmia may be difficult to distinguish from sinus or atrial tachycardia. Whenever the origin of the tachycardia cannot be determined, and the QRS complex appears normal, the term **supraventricular tachycardia** is used.

As with other fast-rate arrhythmias, this inefficient rhythm puts stress on the heart and may cause angina, congestive heart failure, or other dangerous conditions. Treatment would be similar to that used for atrial tachycardias.

Wandering pacemaker

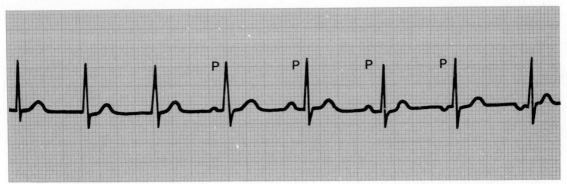

Wandering pacemaker is characterized by shifting sites of impulse formation including the SA node, and atrial and junctional tissue.

The P waves and PR interval may change from beat to beat depending on the pacemaker site. The rhythm is somewhat irregular. The QRS remains normal.

Wandering pacemaker will probably not produce symptoms; it may appear when there is no other evidence of cardiac disease. However, it may be associated with ischemia, inflammation, and digitalis effects. Usually, no treatment is necessary.

HOW TO READ AN ECG

PART III

Ventricular arrhythmias

Ventricular tissue becomes more excitable as a result of ischemia, drug effect, or electrolyte imbalance. Arrhythmias originating in the ventricles may diminish the ability of the heart to function as a pump. Without adequate blood flow, all body organs deteriorate. Quick intervention is vital to correct certain ventricular arrhythmias.

Premature ventricular contractions (PVCs) occur in most MI patients and are the most common and easily recognized rhythm disturbances seen on the ECG. They are also seen in normal persons, caused by smoking, coffee, or alcohol. When pathological, they are seen most often in patients with arteriosclerotic heart disease.

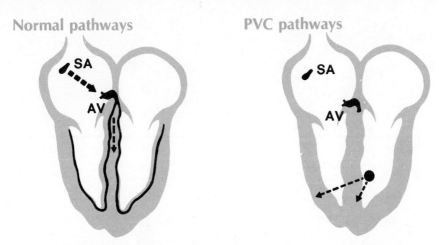

Normal and PVC pathways. As the name denotes, PVCs originate in the ventricles below the AV node. Because the PVCs do not follow the normal conduction path in the ventricles, they show a bizarre QRS configuration on the ECG.

ECG for PVCs

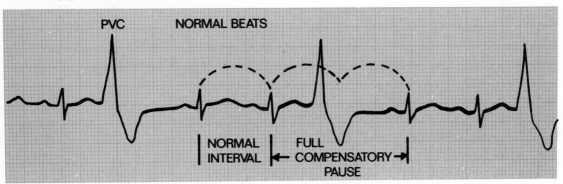

ECG for PVCs. Notice that the PVCs come early in the cycle (premature) and are wider than the normal beat.

Characteristics of PVCs

PVCs can be identified because they:
    1. Occur early in the cycle.
    2. Are not preceded by a P wave.
    3. Have a wide and distorted QRS.
    4. Have a T wave opposite in direction to that of the QRS.
    5. Are usually followed by a full compensatory pause. (The interval between the R waves before and after the PVC is twice that of the normal R-R interval.)

Unifocal PVCs. Those which originate from the same site and therefore have the same configuration.

Multifocal PVCs. Those which originate from different sites and have different shapes.

ECG for multifocal PVCs

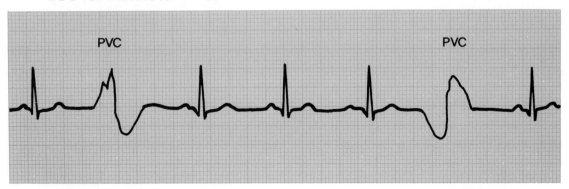

Bigeminy. Paired or coupled rhythm; a repeating pattern of 2 beats, with PVCs and normal beats alternating.

Trigeminy. Rhythm with a repeating pattern of 3 beats; the ratio of PVCs to normal beats is 2:1 or 1:2.

Interpolated PVCs. Those which fall between two normal beats without interrupting the rhythm. This PVC is not followed by a compensatory pause.

ECG for interpolated PVC

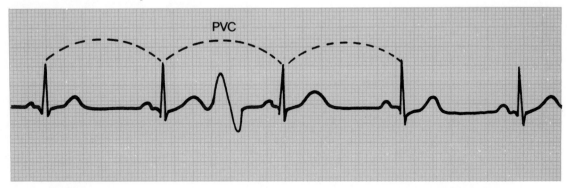

For the patient with an infarct, premature ventricular contractions are usually given vigorous treatment because they can precipitate ventricular fibrillation by hitting a T wave. They are especially dangerous when they:

1. Occur more frequently than one in 10 beats.
2. Occur in groups of two or three.

3. Are landing near the T wave.

4. Take on multiple configurations, since this means that they are coming from different foci, and that the ventricle is more irritable.

"Vigorous treatment" consists of giving lidocaine (Xylocaine), as outlined in the next section on ventricular tachycardia. When PVCs are seen with a normal cardiac rate of over 60 per minute, lidocaine (a suppressant) is the drug of choice because the PVCs are most likely coming from an irritable focus such as ischemic tissue.

On the other hand, if sinus bradycardia occurs (cardiac rate below 60) following a myocardial infarction that involves the SA node, lidocaine is contraindicated. This is why: The PVCs may be occurring as a compensatory mechanism to maintain a reasonable heart rate so as to provide some cardiac contraction and thus pump blood to the body tissues. (The PVCs do not pump as much blood as normal impulses from the SA node, but do provide some circulation.) If the PVCs in this type of bradycardia are not landing on the T wave—which could trigger ventricular fibrillation—atropine is given rather than lidocaine. The atropine increases the rate of the slow-firing SA node, and this terminates the inefficient ectopic beats by replacing them with normal impulses. The usual treatment is 0.6-1.0 mg. of atropine given I.V.

Ventricular tachycardia. This dreaded complication of a myocardial infarct may be defined as a series of multiple (three or more), consecutive PVCs occurring at a rate usually between 150 to 200 per minute. Ventricular tachycardia is very dangerous because it leads to **reduced** cardiac output and, many times, to ventricular fibrillation.

Normal pathways   Ventricular tachycardia pathways

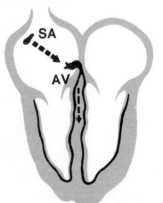 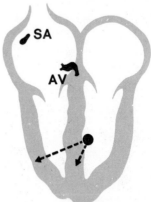

Normal and ventricular tachycardia pathways. These are the same sketches used to illustrate the PVC pathway since ventricular tachycardia can be considered as a series of PVCs. Like the PVCs, the tachycardia shows a bizarre configuration on the ECG.

28

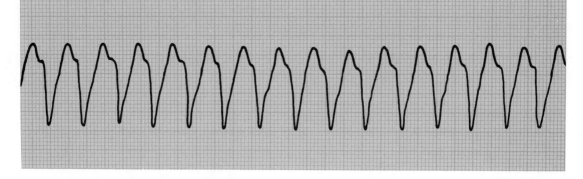

ECG for ventricular tachycardia. Notice that the rate is fast and that the QRS is wide. (A width of three small blocks or more is considered abnormal.) If the ventricular rate is not too fast, independent P waves may sometimes be visible in the QRS complex. (P waves are not shown in this example.)

If the patient is tolerating this arrhythmia fairly well, 75-100 mg. of I.V. lidocaine may be given as a bolus over a two-minute period, repeated in two or three minutes, if necessary. If this is effective, a continuous I.V. drip of lidocaine should be started, delivering 1-3 mg. per minute. The concentration of lidocaine in 5% glucose in water will depend on the patient's tolerance of I.V. fluid.

If the concentration results in too much fluid for the patient, the amount of lidocaine should be increased in the solution. When the heart muscle already is weakened, the cardiac patient should not receive excessive fluid because this may precipitate congestive failure. ("Congestive failure" means that the heart cannot pump all the fluid presented to it, and the result is stasis of the blood in the lungs and other body tissues.)

If lidocaine is ineffective and the patient with ventricular tachycardia loses consciousness, countershock should be instituted. Lidocaine should follow, as delineated above, for at least 24 hours.

Ventricular fibrillation. It is extremely important to be cognizant of this rhythm, for the first qualified person to see the patient should institute therapy immediately. If the arrhythmia is not terminated, the patient will die within minutes.

Normal and ventricular fibrillation pathways. In the fibrillating heart, it can be considered that numerous ectopic foci in the ventricles are firing simultaneously. Thus, there is no effective contraction of the cardiac musculature, and the patient has no pulse.

Normal pathways	Ventricular fibrillation pathways

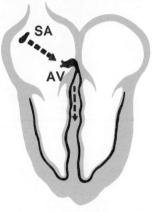 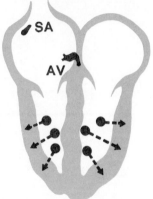

ECG for ventricular fibrillation

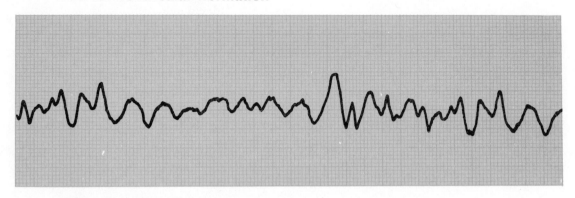

ECG for ventricular fibrillation. Notice the complete distortion and irregularity of the complexes. Similar distortion may also be caused by the movement of the patient or the monitor wires, so it is important to rule out these possibilities. If the patient is alert, or if not alert and has a pulse, the rhythm is **not** ventricular fibrillation. There is no pulse in ventricular fibrillation.

PVC causing ventricular fibrillation

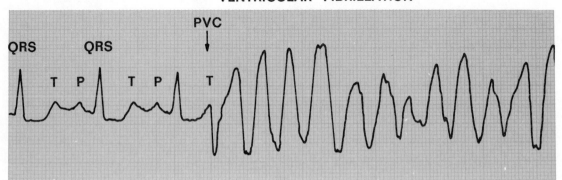

PVC causing ventricular fibrillation. When a PVC lands near the peak of the T wave (vulnerable period), it may precipitate fibrillation as shown. This ECG also illustrates why electrical defibrillation is necessary rather than cardioversion, which may be used to stop other arrhythmias. In cardioversion, a synchronized electrical shock is timed so that it does not hit the T wave; otherwise the heart might go into ventricular fibrillation. In defibrillation, the electrical shock fires immediately, for there are no T waves in ventricular fibrillation.

For adults, an electrical shock of 400 watt-seconds is given with the defibrillator; for children, an initial shock of 200 watt-seconds may be given. The purpose is to stop the heart and allow the SA node to resume normal conduction.

ECG of a successful defibrillation

| VENTRICULAR FIBRILLATION | ELECTRICAL DEFIBRILLATION | EFFECTIVE HEARTBEAT |

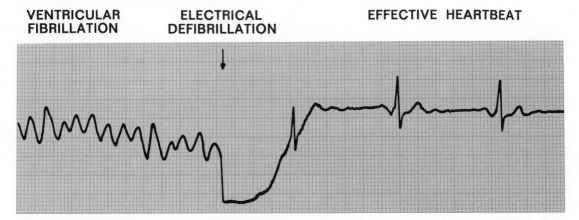

ECG of a successful defibrillation. Clearly shown is the point at which the electrical shock stopped the fibrillating heart. After a moment, it began to beat in normal fashion.

Idioventricular rhythm appears when all complexes originate from the ventricles (wide, distorted, identical QRSs), which occurs when there is no adequate atrial pacemaker, or when the impulse is blocked at the AV node. The rate corresponds to that of ventricular pacemakers (usually below 40).

The patient with this condition requires close observation and may be treated depending on the underlying pathology.

Accelerated idioventricular rhythm (or slow ventricular tachycardia) is another term used to indicate an arrhythmia originating from the ventricle. The rate is usually from 60-100. The QRS complexes are broad, and this rhythm is preceded or followed by a fusion beat. Accelerated idioventricular rhythm, which may occur in an acute MI, comes and goes spontaneously. It does not necessarily predispose to

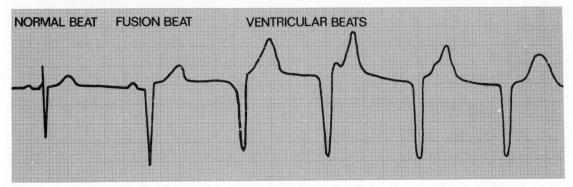

NORMAL BEAT   FUSION BEAT   VENTRICULAR BEATS

the development of fast ventricular tachycardia or ventricular fibrillation and does not require treatment.

Ventricular standstill occurs when the ventricles do not initiate any
backup rhythm in the absence of impulses conducted from the atria. If
this happens with complete heart block, only P waves will be seen. In
the absence of atrial pacemakers, the monitor will show a straight line.

There will be no QRS complexes, and the patient will have no pulse.
Emergency resuscitation measures must be instituted immediately.

AV block

In this condition the AV node is diseased and has difficulty conducting
the P waves into the ventricles. The most common causes are arteriosclerosis and myocardial infarction.

AV block

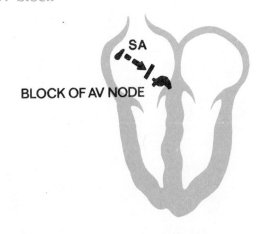

SA

BLOCK OF AV NODE

AV block. Scarring, inflammation, or edema prevents or slows transmission of the electrical impulse by the AV node. The degree of block varies from very slight to complete and is classified as first, second, or third degree block.

First degree AV block

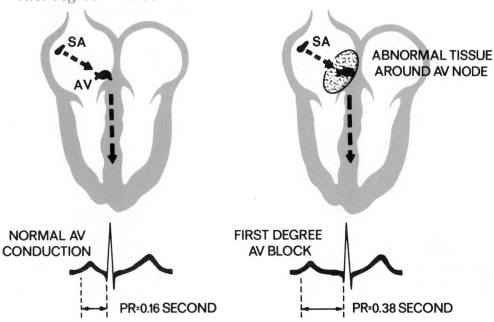

First degree AV block. Because the tissue around the AV node is abnormal, the impulse takes longer to traverse the area.

This is reflected by an increased length in the PR interval on the ECG. (The PR interval represents the impulse going through the atrium and the area of the AV node.) In contrast to second and third degree blocks, all P waves in first degree block penetrate the ventricles to form QRS complexes. In normal conduction, the PR interval is not over 0.20 second (five small blocks on the ECG paper where each block equals 0.04 second). A PR interval such as the one shown (0.38 second) is an indication of first degree block.

First degree block does not diminish cardiac output. However, it is an indicator of possible damage to junctional tissue or of drug effect, especially from digitalis. Observe carefully for possible progression to higher degrees of block.

Second degree AV block exists when some of the P waves are conducted to the ventricles and others are blocked at the AV node. This condition is divided into two classifications: Mobitz I (Wenckebach) and Mobitz II.

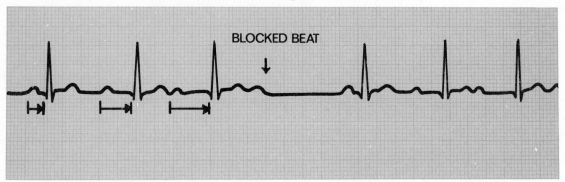

BLOCKED BEAT

Mobitz I (Wenckebach). The ischemic or drug-affected AV node requires a progressively longer interval of time to transmit each beat until a beat fails to be conducted. When the next impulse arrives, the rested AV node is able to transmit the beat in a normal time, but the PR interval again lengthens, and the cycle repeats.

On the ECG, this results in a progressive lengthening of the PR interval until a beat is blocked (P not followed by a QRS) and then the cycle repeats. The rhythm (R-R interval) is irregular, and there are more P waves than QRS complexes.

Wenckebach block may be caused by digitalis or MI, especially one involving the inferior wall. It is generally transient and reversible.

Observe the patient for an excessively slow ventricular rate. If treatment is required, atropine or isoproterenol (Isuprel) are the drugs commonly used to speed the heart rate. Insertion of a pacemaker generally is not necessary.

Mobitz II second degree block

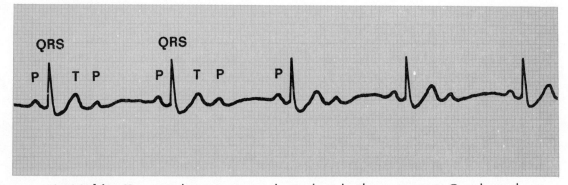

QRS   QRS

P   T   P   P   T   P   P

In **Mobitz II,** some beats are conducted and others are not. Conducted beats have a consistent PR interval. In blocked beats, there is a P wave not followed by a QRS complex.

One type of pattern shows a specific ratio of blocked beats such as 2:1, 3:1, or 4:1. In such cases, the R-R interval will be regular.

The example shows a 2:1 second degree block. Every second P wave is conducted to the ventricles.

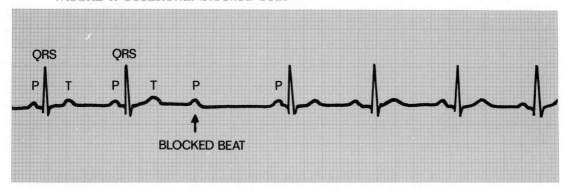

Mobitz II occasional blocked beat. Another pattern presents as an occasional nonconducted P wave. In this case, the blocked P will occur at the expected cycle interval.

One consequence of Mobitz II can be a slow ventricular rate resulting in low cardiac output. This diminished output can produce myocardial or cerebral ischemia. Early indications of cerebral insufficiency include mental confusion, dullness, or agitation.

Mobitz II is more likely than Mobitz I to progress to a greater degree of block. Thus, to treat Mobitz II, many cardiologists insert a pacemaker that is activated when the cardiac rate falls.

To increase the heart rate while awaiting pacemaker insertion, .06-1.0 mg. atropine I.V. may be given. If the rate cannot be maintained with atropine, 1.0 mg. isoproterenol (Isuprel) in 250 cc. of 5% glucose in water may be infused.

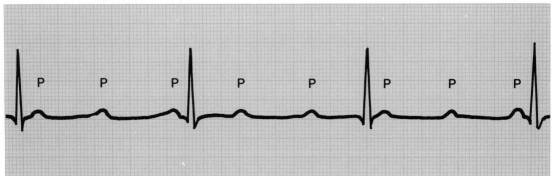

Third degree AV block is also called complete heart block. In this arrhythmia, no atrial impulses (P waves) activate the ventricles. The QRS originates from a junctional or ventricular pacemaker site. There-

fore, the P waves and QRS complexes occur independently.

Both the P waves and QRS complexes occur regularly, but there is no relationship between them. The PR interval varies and some P waves may be partly obscured by QRS complexes.

Complete heart block may be caused by inflammation, scarring, myocardial infarction, or drugs such as digitalis. The pulse rate is usually slow because of the inherent rate of junctional or ventricular pacemaker sites. Since these secondary pacemakers are not dependable, the treatment of choice is an artificial pacemaker. Isoproterenol (Isuprel) may be given to increase the ventricular rate while awaiting insertion of a transvenous pacemaker. While administering isoproterenol, watch the monitor for the appearance of frequent PVCs or ventricular tachycardia. Atropine would not be effective because it increases only the atrial rate.

Conduction delays in AV blocks

AV block	Impulses	Rhythm	PR interval	ECG
First degree	All conducted (with delay)	Regular	Prolonged (>0.20 sec.); constant	
Second degree Mobitz I (Wenckebach)	Some conducted, some blocked	Irregular	Progressively longer until dropped beat; cyclic pattern	
Second degree Mobitz II	Some conducted, some blocked	Irregular	Constant for conducted beats; some Ps without QRSs; can appear 2:1, 3:1, or occasionally	
Third degree	None conducted	Regular QRS; independent regular P	Variable; no P-QRS relationship	

Artificial pacemaker

An artificial pacemaker uses a pulse generator (power source) to stimulate the myocardium and produce a ventricular contraction. The power is delivered to the endocardium through a transvenous pacing catheter threaded into the right ventricle. Another way to stimulate the myocardium is through small electrodes sewn onto the surface of the heart, but it requires a thoracotomy and is rarely used.

A pacemaker may be indicated when natural pacemaker activity ceases or the heart does not maintain a sufficiently rapid rate. Arrhythmias resulting in slow rates include bradycardia that does not respond to drug therapy, and heart block with a slow ventricular response.

Pacemakers are sometimes used to overdrive (capture and convert) fast rate arrhythmias. Prophylactic implantation may be done for patients with arrhythmias that may progress to inadequate rates during surgery, or when depressant drugs are being administered. Pacemakers may also be useful for stress testing in patients whose physical conditions contraindicate testing by the usual physical activity.

Transvenous pacemaker

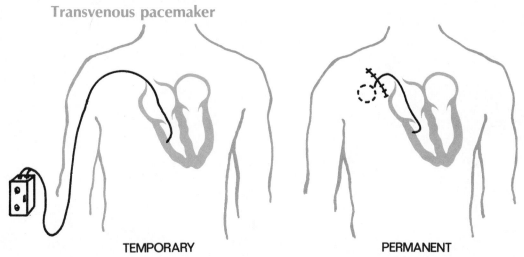

TEMPORARY   PERMANENT

A **temporary pacemaker** uses a transvenous catheter attached to an external pulse generator (power source). It can be inserted quickly using fluoroscopy or ECG feedback for positioning.

For a **permanent pacemaker,** the pulse generator (enclosed in nonreactive plastic) is surgically implanted in superficial muscle tissue. The pacemaker function must be evaluated periodically, and the unit is replaced when necessary. Batteries usually last from 18 months to 3 years. Lithium and nuclear pulse generators last much longer.

The **demand pacemaker** discharges only if the pacemaker does not

sense a natural impulse within a preset time interval. This is the preferred method since it avoids competition between paced and natural beats.

A **fixed rate pacemaker** is not designed to sense the patient's natural beat and fires at a constant, preset rate. It is useful only when the patient has no spontaneous ventricular contraction.

Competition occurs when the pacemaker fires in spite of the patient's natural beat. It is especially dangerous when the impulse occurs during the vulnerable period of the cardiac cycle (the T wave).

The pacemaker artifact (blip) is the ECG indication that an impulse has been fired. It appears as a small vertical line above or below the baseline. If the electrode tip of the catheter is imbedded in the ventricle, the blip will be followed immediately by a wide QRS (similar to a beat originating in the ventricle).

Normally functioning artificial pacemaker

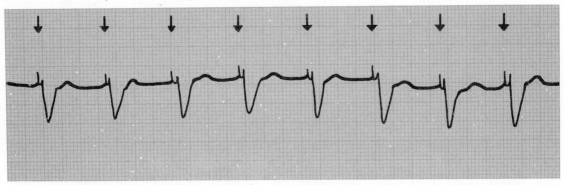

Normally functioning artificial pacemaker. The ECG of a patient with a normally functioning artificial pacemaker shows a small vertical line (see arrows) at the beginning of each QRS complex. This line represents the electrical stimulus of the artificial pacemaker.

Malfunctioning pacemaker

PACEMAKER BEATS   ABSENCE OF PACEMAKER BEATS

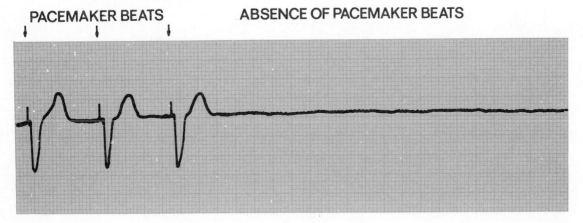

Malfunctioning pacemaker. This situation is easily recognized by noting that the vertical pacemaker beats shown on the ECG cease and the heartbeats stop. Common causes of pacemaker malfunction or failure are breakage of the wires from pacemaker to heart, disconnection of these wires at the pacemaker, and battery failure. When a battery runs down, the pacing rate may be faster or slower than the preset rate. The pacemaker function, including battery life, should be checked periodically using equipment designed for this purpose.

Non-capture (no contact between pacemaker and heart)

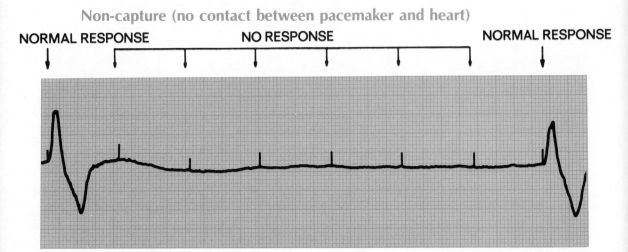

NORMAL RESPONSE   NO RESPONSE   NORMAL RESPONSE

Non-capture (no contact between pacemaker and heart). This is one of the most common causes of pacing failure. It occurs when the wires from the pacemaker pull loose from the heart wall, usually as a result of the patient's sudden movement. It is readily identified on the ECG. The QRS complex that normally follows the pacemaker stimulus (arrow at left) suddenly disappears. It resumes (right) when contact is made again. Notice that the small vertical line of the pacemaker stimulus continues, indicating that the pacemaker is functioning but without contact with the heart wall.

HOW TO READ AN ECG

PART IV
Miscellaneous rhythm disturbances   Page 40
Identification of MI   Page 46
ECG changes in stress testing   Page 48

Miscellaneous rhythm disturbances

This section contains definitions and brief descriptions of other more complicated arrhythmias encountered in ECG monitoring. Additional information about these subjects can be found in comprehensive electrocardiography textbooks.

ECG for fusion beat

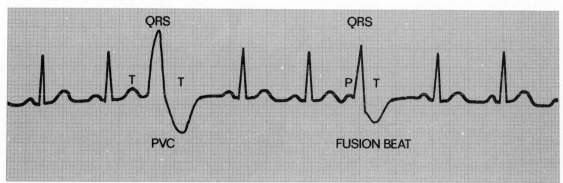

A **fusion beat** results when an impulse from the sinus node activates the atria just when an ectopic ventricular impulse discharges. This coincidence produces a P wave before a wide QRS complex in which the QRS is partly normal and partly like a ventricular beat.

A fusion beat may appear as a single beat, or it may initiate a run of ventricular beats or ventricular tachycardia.

ECG for capture beat

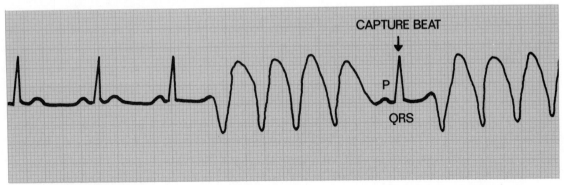

A **capture beat** is an impulse that takes control of the heartbeat. For example: A ventricular capture beat is conducted from another area to "capture" the ventricles.

During an episode of ventricular tachycardia, the atria continue to function independently. Occasionally, an atrial impulse occurs when the ventricles can respond. This one beat, conducted through the ventricles in a normal fashion, results in a normal complex in the midst of a run of ventricular tachycardia.

Capture also refers to an ectopic pacemaker, or to a beat generated by an artificial pacemaker.

ECG for escape beat (junctional)

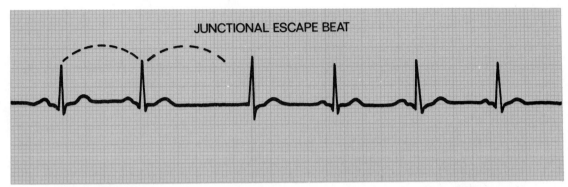

An **escape beat** may occur after a pause longer than the usual R-R interval. It originates in junctional or ventricular tissue and functions as part of the heart's backup pacing system to prevent cardiac arrest. It

compensates for a lapse in sinus node activity. If a conducted rhythm does not resume, this escape beat may initiate a continuing rhythm.

ECG for blocked PAC

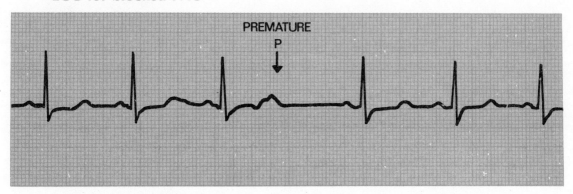

PREMATURE
P

Blocked premature atrial contraction (PAC). A blocked PAC occurs when an irritable focus in the atria fires a premature impulse that depolarizes atrial tissue; the impulse is not conducted to the ventricles. At this early point in the cycle, the AV node and ventricular tissue are refractory (cannot respond) because they have not yet been repolarized following the previous beat. On the ECG, this appears as a premature P wave not followed by a QRS complex.

Note that the P wave (sometimes buried in the T wave of the previous beat) is premature. It is important to differentiate this blocked PAC from the Mobitz II, which shows an occasional blocked beat (P not premature), and from sinus arrest (no P). The most common reason for a pause in sinus rhythm is a blocked PAC. Blocked PACs may be present in normal hearts, or may occur because of digitalis toxicity or heart disease.

Bundle branch block is an obstruction in the right or left ventricular conduction pathway. When this occurs, the impulse travels first through the unobstructed branch and is then transmitted by nonspecialized myocardial tissue to the opposite ventricle. This aberrant pathway requires a longer time for activation of the ventricles, and the resulting QRS is greater than 0.12 sec. (three small squares). Origin of this beat is from the atria—usually, the SA node. Therefore, a P wave will precede the wide QRS.

Bundle branch block may occur in a single premature beat, because either the right or left branch has not yet been repolarized. It may occur when the rate becomes too fast to permit adequate repolarization between beats (rate-dependent). It may also result from disease or ischemia in this part of the conduction system.

To determine which bundle branch is blocked, we must look at Lead V_1 or Modified Chest Lead I (MCL$_1$). From this viewpoint on the right

side of the heart, we can observe the direction of current flow.

When the **right bundle branch** is blocked, the impulse travels first through the left ventricle (upward deflection or R wave), and then activates the right ventricle (second upward deflection or R'). This produces an M-shaped complex in V₁ or MCL₁.

If the entire **left bundle branch** is blocked, the impulse first depolarizes the right side of the heart and then—through aberrant pathways—the left ventricle, producing a wide, deep V-shaped complex. A small, upright R may appear before this complex.

Right bundle branch block   Left bundle branch block

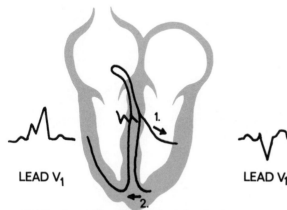

LEAD V₁

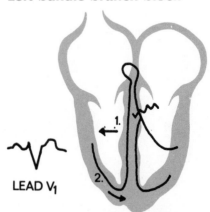

LEAD V₁

Right bundle branch block is more common because the right branch is a long, narrow pathway. The left bundle branch is thicker at its origin and subdivides into anterior superior and posterior inferior branches. When one of these subdivisions (fascicles) becomes blocked, it is called a hemiblock, or monofascicular block. It does not produce a QRS greater than 0.12 sec., and is diagnosed by axis determination. When the right bundle branch and either fascicle of the left bundle become blocked, it is called bifascicular block.

Conduction pathway—hemiblock

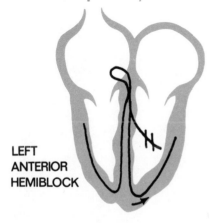

LEFT
ANTERIOR
HEMIBLOCK

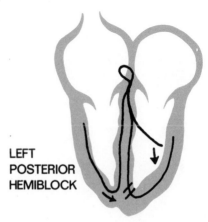

LEFT
POSTERIOR
HEMIBLOCK

Bundle branch block can occur in healthy hearts and in a variety of disease conditions. Additional data is required to determine its significance. Cardiac depressant drugs should be used with caution because they can aggravate the conduction delay.

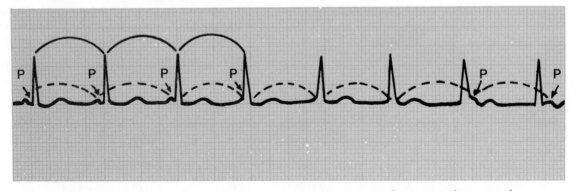

A-V dissociation exists whenever separate pacemakers simultaneously control the atria and ventricles. Two separate sites send impulses, and independent rhythms coexist to pace the upper and lower chambers.

The term A-V dissociation is used by different authors to describe a variety of conduction disturbances. The following are some of the more widely recognized variations:

A-V dissociation can exist because of an inadequate atrial pacemaker. For example: When impulses from the sinus node or atria are excessively slow, pacemakers from the junctional or ventricular areas interpose escape beats or rhythms.

When the atrial pacemaker impulse is intermittently blocked from the ventricles, separate atrial and junctional or ventricular rhythms may be established. These rhythms may have almost identical rates.

Irritability in an ectopic site may result in a rapid junctional or ventricular rhythm. A separate atrial rhythm coexists. For example: ventricular tachycardia with unrelated P waves.

ECG for Wolff-Parkinson-White (WPW)

NORMAL COMPLEX   WPW   COMPLEX

DELTA WAVE

Wolff-Parkinson-White (WPW) syndrome. A pre-excitation syndrome exists when atrial impulses are transmitted directly to the ventricles through shortcut conduction pathways. The impulses do not travel

44

through the AV node and thus avoid the normal conduction delay that occurs there.

The syndrome carries the names of those physicians who described one atypical conduction pattern. The ECG is characterized by:
1. A short PR interval (less than .12)
2. A slurred upstroke on the QRS (delta wave)
3. A wide QRS (greater than .12)
4. Secondary ST and T wave changes (depolarization is altered)

The mechanism of WPW is thought to be the utilization of a highly developed branch of the conduction system called the bundle of Kent. This connects the conduction system of the atria to either ventricle, bypassing the AV node. This could occur on either the left (type A) or right (type B) side of the heart.

Individuals afflicted with this condition are subject to episodes of supraventricular tachycardia. This arrhythmia may be resistant to the usual treatment for PAT. It is important to differentiate it from ventricular tachycardia and other arrhythmias with wide QRS complexes.

Effect of drugs and electrolytes on the ECG. Changes in the shape of the ECG complex may result from presence or absence of certain substances that influence myocardial tissue. Here are the most common, showing their ECG effect.

Agent	Effect on myocardium	ECG change	Example
Hypokalemia (low serum potassium)	Increases irritability (ectopic beats)	Decreases height of T wave; produces U wave	
Hyperkalemia (high serum potassium)	Depresses automaticity (standstill)	Creates tall, peaked T waves; prolongs PR interval	
Hypocalcemia (low serum calcium)	Decreases threshold for stimulation	Prolongs Q-T interval	
Hypercalcemia (high serum calcium)	Increases threshold for stimulation	Shortens Q-T interval	
Digitalis	Depresses conduction; increases automaticity (predisposes to many arrhythmias)	Produces downward deflection of S-T segment; prolongs PR interval	
Quinidine	Depresses conduction and automaticity	Widens QRS; prolongs PR interval	

Many additional drugs, such as antiarrhythmics and tranquilizers, can change the ECG pattern. Drugs need not reach toxic blood levels to produce ECG changes.

Identification of MI

One of the most significant uses of a 12-lead ECG is determining a myocardial infarction. The physician locates the damage by noting which leads show indicative changes. (You may recall that Leads II, III, and AVF show the inferior or diaphragmatic area of the heart. The precordial or chest leads reflect changes on the anterior surface.) Many factors can influence the 12-lead ECG interpretation. Changes most characteristic of an MI are presented in the following section.

One important point to remember about the ECG interpretation of MI is that about 15 per cent of infarcts show no changes on the initial tracing. Therefore, if a person has symptoms compatible with a heart attack and has a normal ECG, he nevertheless should be admitted to the hospital for observation and further electrocardiograms.

The usual first finding in an infarct is elevation of the ST segment. This is followed by T wave inversion, which in turn is followed by a large Q wave. As the infarct heals, the Q wave may remain as the only sign of an old coronary occlusion. This is the sequence:

Sequence of the ECG following MI

Sequence of the ECG following MI. (1) Normal. (2) Hours after infarction, the ST segment becomes elevated. (3) Hours to days later, the T wave inverts and the Q wave becomes larger. (4) Days to weeks later, the ST segment returns to near-normal. (5) Weeks to months later, the T wave becomes upright again, but the Q wave may remain large.

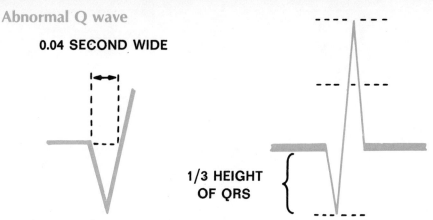

0.04 SECOND WIDE

1/3 HEIGHT OF QRS

Abnormal Q wave. Since a large Q wave is many times indicative of an old infarction (except in AVR where a large Q wave is normal), the question is often asked how large a Q wave can be before it is considered abnormal. A Q wave may be considered abnormal if it is over 0.04 second wide (one small block on the ECG paper), or if it is greater in depth than one-third the height of the QRS complex.

In summary: A fresh myocardial infarction is characterized by ST elevation and T wave inversion. An enlarged Q wave is indicative of an old infarction.

Inferior wall infarction

I	AVR	V1-2
II	AVL	V3-4
III	AVF	V5-6

Inferior wall infarction. Very early pattern showing ST elevation in Leads II, III, and AVF.

Anterior wall infarction

I	AVR	V1-2
II	AVL	V3-4
III	AVF	V5-6

Anterior wall infarction. Later pattern (many hours to a few days) showing Q waves and T wave inversion in Leads I, AVL, and V3-6.

ECG changes in stress testing

An ECG of the resting heart does not predict a myocardial infarction. Unfortunately, some people have shown normal ECGs during a routine physical exam, only to suffer a fatal heart attack shortly thereafter.

An ECG recorded during periods of physical activity may be a more accurate indicator of factors that could predispose to a myocardial infarction. Reason: As the heart rate increases, the myocardium needs more oxygen, and narrow coronary arteries will not provide a sufficient oxygen supply.

Before testing, the candidate is examined by the physician; pertinent cardiopulmonary data, including a resting ECG, are recorded. The patient is stressed by having him expend measured amounts of energy on a calibrated exercise device such as a treadmill or an ergometer (exercise bicycle). During the activity, a continuous ECG tracing and other vital signs are monitored.

Indicators of myocardial ischemia are ST depression or ST elevation. Some patients will develop anginal pain during periods of myocardial hypoxia, and others will not. If a person has typical anginal pain and negative ECG changes, the test is still considered positive. Extraventricular systoles or other arrhythmias may indicate a positive test.

The following diagram shows some possible ST segment changes under stress:

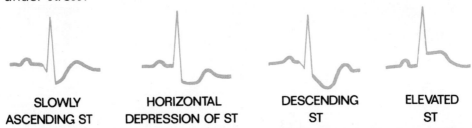

| SLOWLY ASCENDING ST | HORIZONTAL DEPRESSION OF ST | DESCENDING ST | ELEVATED ST |

Information obtained through this test serves to indicate the extent of coronary artery disease.

Other tests which can amplify information about the heart include vectorcardiograms, echocardiograms, and phonocardiograms. Radioisotope scans and cardiac catheterization provide additional diagnostic details about the heart's structure and function.

Summary of basic arrhythmias

Type of arrhythmia	Appearance of ECG	Characteristic abnormality	Conduction pathway
Normal rhythm			
Sinus arrhythmia		Irregular rhythm	
Sinus tachycardia		Rate 100-150	
Sinus bradycardia		Rate below 60	
PACs		Premature P; normal QRS	
PAT		Rate 140-250	
Atrial flutter		Saw-toothed flutter waves	
Atrial fibrillation		No clearly defined P; irregular rhythm	
Junctional rhythm		Inverted or hidden P	
JPCs		Premature beat; inverted or hidden P; normal QRS	
PVCs		Premature beat; no P; wide, distorted QRS	
Ventricular tachycardia		Series of PVCs; rate 150-200	

Type of arrhythmia	Appearance of ECG	Characteristic abnormality	Conduction pathway
Ventricular fibrillation	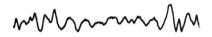	No well-defined complexes	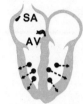
First degree heart block	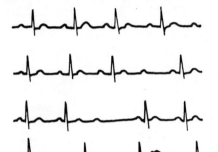	PR greater than 0.20; constant PR	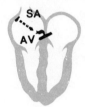
Second degree Mobitz I (Wenckebach)		Progressively longer PR until dropped beat; cyclic pattern	
Second degree Mobitz II		Some nonconducted Ps (2:1, 3:1, or occasional); constant PR	
Third degree complete heart block		No relationship between P and QRS	

Index